Graves' Disease Secrets

Jen Daniele

www.GravesRecoveryCamp.com

Copyright © 2019 by Jen Daniele

All rights reserved.

No part of this publication may be reproduced, distributed, or transmitted in any form or by any means, including photocopying, recording, or other electronic or mechanical methods, without the prior written permission of the publisher, except in the case of brief quotations embodied in critical reviews and certain other noncommercial uses permitted by copyright law. For permission requests, write to the publisher, addressed "Attention: Permissions Coordinator," at the address below.
Disclaimer: The material presented here is for informational purposes only. As each individual situation is unique, you should use proper discretion, in consultation with a health care practitioner, before undertaking the protocols, diet, exercises, techniques, or otherwise described herein. The author and publisher expressly disclaim responsibility for any adverse effects that may result from the use or application of the information contained herein.

ISBN: 9781099581755

DEDICATION

I dedicate this book to my loving husband Bobby and my kids Charlie, Audrey and Owen.

CONTENTS

About the Author

1. Introduction
2. What is Hyperthyroidism & Graves' Disease
3. Hyperthyroidism Symptoms
4. Types of Treatments
5. Establishing your Healthcare Team
6. Working with Your Healthcare Team
7. Types of Tests
8. How to Approach Your Mind
9. Healthy Habits
10. Believe You Can Heal Your Body

About the Author

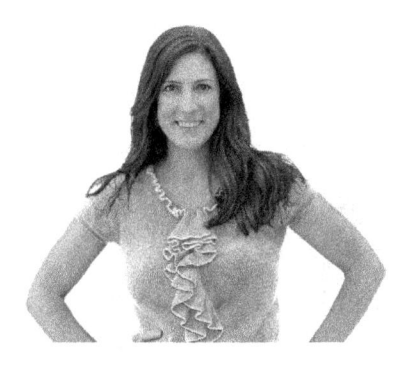

Hi, my name is Jen, and I wanted to welcome you to my labor of love. It looks like a book but here's the story.

You see, I grew up in Oregon and didn't realize I was in the hotbed for all-natural living. I just took it for granted that everyone wanted fresh milk from the guy down the street.

Since then I've juiced my own wheatgrass and today we have a sprouter going all the time growing fresh sprouts in the house.

My goal was to always be healthy.

My Story...

So, I told you before that I am a health food enthusiast. I was a competitive gymnast for 10 years and was always the epitome of health.

That all changed when I went to the dentist as an adult and the hygienist found a lump on my neck.

Yes, I was nervous to say the least. I was diagnosed with Hyperthyrodism and Graves' disease.

Self-Help Nut...

In high school I was always getting positive thinking books. I became addicted to reading new age psychology and I loved it. I was intrigued at how we could control our own path by controlling that piece of meat that is in between my ears!

I used a lot of what I learned and applied it to my gymnastics. So many of the tricks we performed, like a back flip on a balance beam were completely safe, but the reason girls didn't try was because of the fear. I learned that if you could make it up in your mind to do something, then your body would do it!

Getting Better

It's taken a long time, but I'm healing naturally from Graves'. If you told me four years ago that I'd be gluten and dairy free, I'd say you were crazy!

I wish I had a community of people who understood what I was going through. It would have been helpful in my journey to be able to ask people how they made such dramatic changes in their lives.

This is why I created GravesRecovery Camp.com. I want people to have a place to go for the support they need to get better.

My body thanks me for the changes I've made and I want to help you make those changes as well. Let's get started!

Chapter 1 – Introduction

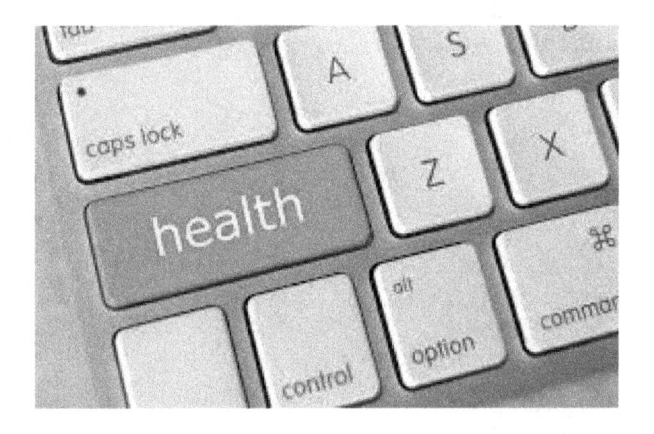

You've got Graves' disease. It can be overwhelming diagnosis. There is so much to figure out about it. Many times people start by asking how did I get it? Why me? Most likely you have had it for a while and the symptoms got so bad that you were finally diagnosed.

It's hard not to worry, but I'm here to tell you that I believe that we may be able to heal ourselves without irreversible medical intervention.

After being diagnosed myself, I learned so much along my Graves' disease recovery journey that I wanted to help others who were in the same situation. When you start researching there is so much differing advice and it is all very difficult to sort out. Some is very technical and scientific that it's hard to understand.

After learning about healing from the inside out, I experienced how overwhelming it is to do all the things you need to do on a consistent basis. It's life changing. It's easy to get depressed and throw in the towel by succumbing to irreversible treatments that have their own permanent side effects. I believe that with the right support people can recover from this disease.

There are many different views on how to treat Graves' depending on the type of physician you see. I recommend engaging both an endocrinologist and a naturopath. You become the liaison and the patient who works with both to generate the best outcome for you.

Becoming your own healthcare advocate can be a daunting task. You are the one taking responsibility for your own health. It is quite an effort to first understand everything that is happening in the doctor visits, remember to do everything that is asked of you and transfer all the information between physicians.

It's also important to consider that

everyone is different too. Not only in your own body, but in their environment and the medical resources you have access to. What works for one person may not work for you. On your road to recovery, you may be hopeful that a certain treatment will work, only to find out that it didn't work for you. At those points it's important to figure out a way to work through it.

As you begin to get treatment, some things may work for you and some may not. You can put your best effort into the ideas that are recommended to you by your doctors. You will learn this new language of autoimmune diseases and Graves' disease.

At some point you won't have to have your blood drawn all the time, you won't be anxiously waiting for test results. But this will take time. It'll take patience, perseverance, and many changes in your life.

The biggest concern for me is to avoid any irreversible treatments. In this book we'll explore the details, but the point is that removing your thyroid for hyperthyroidism results in hypothyroidism 80% of the time. Once you have taken out your thyroid, you'll be dealing with your thyroid for the rest of your life.

This book will give you a fresh perspective on mobilizing the resources you need. I'll give you ideas on how to approach balancing the care you will receive from conventional and alternative medical treatments.

If you need more one-on-one help and consistent support encouragement like I did, please join the GravesRecoveryCamp.com community. If you have any questions, please just email me at jen@gravesrecoverycamp.com.

Chapter 2 – What is Graves' Disease

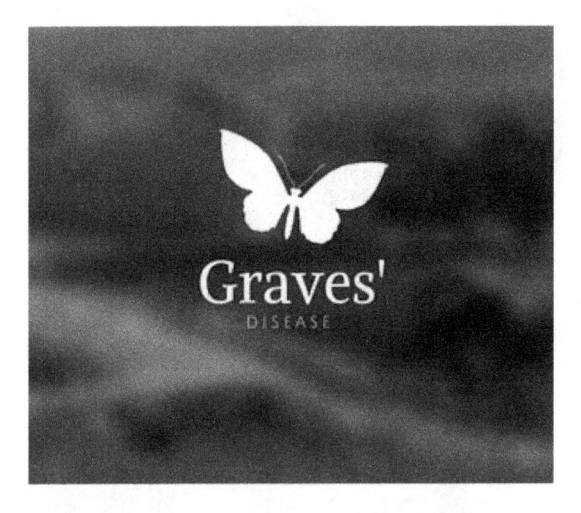

There are many things about this disease that I don't like and the first thing is the name. Graves' Disease. Sounds so morbid, it's just an unfortunate name.

The reason it's called Graves' is because Robert James Graves discovered the disease. It's a bit controversial that he was the first person to discover it, he just had a better publicist over 150 years ago than the Carl A. von Basedow who had researched the disease five years before Graves'. So, we're stuck with Graves' instead of Basedow.

What we know now, is that there are several types of hyperthyroidism, each associated with a different specific cause. The most common type of hyperthyroidism is Graves' Disease.

In Graves' disease, your immune system creates antibodies known as thyroid-stimulating immunoglobulins. These antibodies then attach to healthy thyroid cells. They can cause your thyroid to create too much thyroid hormone.

The thyroid is usually regulated by areas of the brain – the pituitary gland and hypothalamus – that tell it to appropriately turn on and off. These antibodies interrupt the normal feedback mechanism that regulates production of right amounts of thyroid hormone, causing levels to be abnormally high.

We still don't know what factors cause the immune system to attack the thyroid gland.

Some believe there may be a genetic component, but it is not proven. Graves' does occur more in women and people over the age of 20.

If left untreated, Graves' may cause weight loss, anxiety, depression, thyroid eye disease and fatigue. I personally was diagnosed with this condition, and had many of the common symptoms associated with it.

Conventional treatment methods include medications like Methimazole and heart medication, or in many cases radioactive iodine treatment or surgery. Alternative treatments focus on healing the immune system, which gets to the root cause of the body attacking itself. These treatments are focused on the whole person and have helped many people recover from the disease.

Chapter 3 – Hyperthyroidism Symptoms

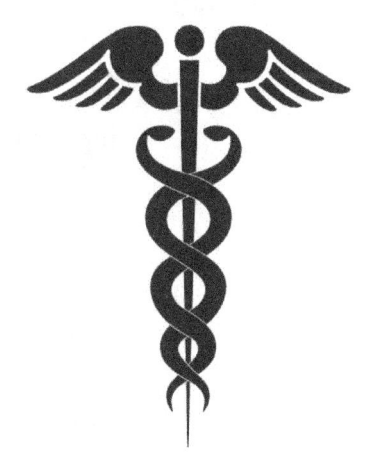

I had the symptoms for Graves' disease long before I was ever diagnosed. I had been extremely hungry all the time, I ate everything in sight, but I didn't gain a thing. I stayed up late, I woke up early. At the time I was a mom three kids under 4 years old and I worked full time at a pretty intense job (or I just took it extremely seriously and made it intense!). I loved having all the energy, but there was something else going on. I was hot all the time, even in the winter. My legs itched and I was extremely shaky. When I read bedtime stories to my kids I got out of breath. I thought it was from coming up the stairs, but I was in shape.

I didn't listen to my body!

It wasn't until I went to the dentist that the hygienist noticed a lump on my neck and suggested I get it checked out. All I could think is that it could be cancer. Then what would I do? I have three kids, I'm not ready to leave them. After a couple months of denial, and trying got to get into an endocrinologist on my own, I went to visit my Primary Care Physician. Since I had a feeling something was going on with my thyroid, I asked for some thyroid blood tests before my appointment.

The tests confirmed that I had Graves', but I hadn't recognized that I had a diagnosable disease!

There are a lot of symptoms associated with Graves' Disease. Here are the most common:

- More than your normal anxiety and irritability.

- Shaking in your hands or fingers, like you've had five cups of coffee!

- Heat sensitivity and an increase in perspiration. I was wearing sleeveless shirts even when there was snow on the ground!

- Weight loss, despite normal eating habits. I was eating everything in sight. I would have snacks all the time and I couldn't stay away from the vending machine at work.

- Enlargement of your thyroid gland. It's called a goiter – not my favorite word in the world. I didn't notice it, but once it was pointed out to me I did notice it.

- Change in menstrual cycles. This is for the ladies. I never kept track of my timing, but I bet if I had, I would have noticed a difference.

- More frequent than usual bowel movements.

- Bulging eyes. The eyes seem to be the signature picture for this disease. It's just so startling to see.

- Thick, red skin usually on the shins or tops of the feet.

- Rapid heartbeat. It feels like your heart is beating hard even though you have not been exercising.

- Changes in your finger nails. Your nails may grow fast, but could be pitted or peel. They may be ragged and brittle. Mine even had more space under the nail between the nail and the skin.

Even though these are the common symptoms of Graves', many people will not experience them especially in the early stages.

When I first started researching the disease, the pictures of people with the bulging eyes really freaked me out. My doctor's assured me that would not happen since we were treating the disease and it was not progressing.

Please don't let all your research scare you. This is a serious disease, but you are taking the steps to manage your health and there are medical treatments for the disease.

Chapter 4 – Types of Treatments

Typically, conventional medicine treats the symptoms not the patient. Thankfully, there have been a lot of people dedicated to figuring out how to address the cause of the disease. They focus on how to reduce the production of the thyroid hormone which minimizes the symptoms. But, treating the symptoms helps you feel more comfortable, which is a relief.

The disease has been diagnosed since the early 1800's. Since the first definitive treatments were developed, like radioactive iodine in 1941, no innovative treatments have been developed.

Here is an overview of each type of traditional treatment.

Radio Active Iodine Therapy

This treatment is pretty scary because you have the radioactivity inside your body and it then can be emitted from your skin. Anything you touch can then have the radioactivity, if anyone in your household touches that item, they can be exposed to the radioactivity as well. When discussing this with my endocrinologist, she suggested that I move into a hotel for a week and not have any interaction with any other person.

Surgery

The thyroid can be removed surgically. Again, this is a definitive treatment. In my opinion, it's much safer than the Radio Active Iodine, but there are all the risks associated with surgery in general. You'll be under anesthesia and you will have a scar on your neck as a result.

Antithyroid Drugs

The last option and least invasive is to take antithyroid medication like methimazole or propylthiouracil. In my experience, most of the endocrinologists I've seen want to move off of the antithyroid drugs, relatively quickly.

The endocrinologists refer to the first

two as Definitive Treatments. That means they are irreversible. Through my research, I have learned that there is an 80% chance that you will then develop Hypothyroidism. If you develop that disease, unfortunately, there isn't much left to do but work closely with your endocrinologist, since your thyroid has been permanently removed and you will be on a hormone replacement.

The risks with these conventional treatments include:

- The medications don't address the underlying cause
- There may be side effects of the medications
- By not treating the underlying cause of the disease, other health issues are likely to develop
- If you remove the thyroid there is no way to get it back!

Thus, in the last 65 years, no additional conventional medical treatments have been developed to address Graves'. It seems as though the medical establishment feels these are effective enough and don't warrant an overhaul. I'm thankful the doctors and researchers have come before to develop these for us, but I think we can address the root cause and really heal.

As various treatments were introduced to me, I knew that I wanted to get healed instead of removing a body part! Remember you are not alone. If you need help figuring out how to stay true to what you want, please email me or join the community GravesRecoveryCamp.com.

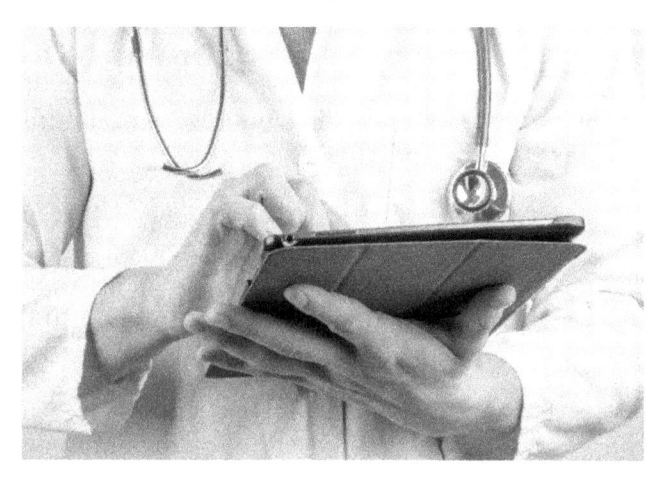

Chapter 5 – Establishing Your Healthcare Team

It's important to put your own team together who can help you get better. The goal of the team is to find the cause and restore your health back to normal.

Remember, self-treating even with natural supplements can actually hurt you. The Graves' disease is the result, not the cause of the problem and you may be focused on thyroid supplements. Other areas can be involved like the adrenals, your gut and other hormones. Having professionals help you navigate these connected systems is extremely critical.

If you can, find an endocrinologist who has experience in treating Grave's disease. You want someone who has experience, not someone who is merely following the protocol, who wants to remove your thyroid.

This may seem easy, but it requires homework up front. Most Endocrinologists want you to be referred to them, even if your insurance does not require a referral. That means you need to interview the Endocrinologists and ask your referring doctor to refer you to a particular doctor.

I ended up visiting a few different endocrinologists for different reasons, one retired, another moved away, one was not compassionate about what I was going through.

The point is, you need a good one, but you may not stay with that one through your whole recovery.

Here are some questions to get you started:

- How long has Dr. Jones been practicing? You want to know that they have some experience.

- How many patients has s/he treated with Grave's disease, what are the results? Here you are trying to determine their philosophy, how long will they treat before recommending definitive treatments, how patient are thy.

- Does Dr. Jones use an online patient system? I found the online system very helpful in communicating with the doctors and it's helpful for having a record of the labwork and appointments.

- Does Dr. Jones work with a Naturopath? Many endocrinologists don't, but you may be surprised to find out that an endocrinologist does. If they do you are in luck!

The next step is to find a Naturopath. Their focus will be on treating you as a whole person considering the physical, mental, emotional, genetic, environmental and social factors effecting you. Locating a naturopath may be a little more difficult depending on where you live in the country. In this case you will also want to interview the Naturopaths prior to making your appointment.

Here are a few questions:

- How long has Dr. Smith been practicing? How many patients has s/he treated with Grave's disease?

You want to find someone with some experience. If you cannot find a naturopath with Grave's disease experience, don't worry. All Naturopath's are treating the whole person, many times our diseases are just different manifestations of the same underlying issues.

- Does Dr. Smith work with Endocrinologists?

You want the Naturopath to be open to working on your health care team. You will most likely be the liaison between the two doctors, but you want them to be open to working with each other.

Realize that you are responsible for your health and the type of care you get. YOU are going to be crucial in your own healing.

You might need help along the way. I'd encourage you to check out the Graves' Recovery community where you can get the support you need to be the glue for your healthcare team. If you have any questions about getting started, please email me at jen@gravesrecoverycamp.com

Chapter 6 – Working with Your Own Healthcare Team

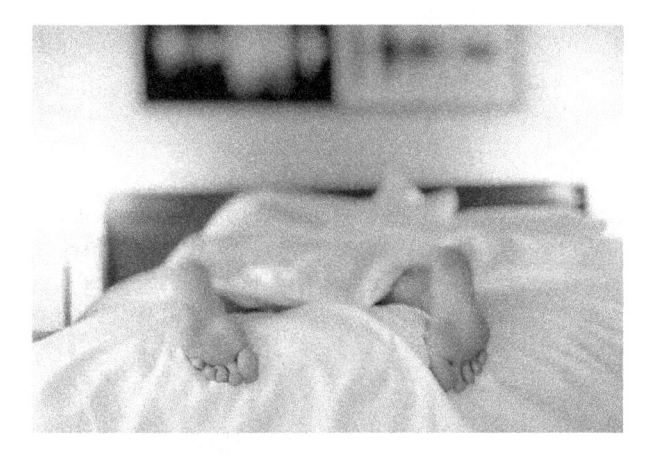

After you have your healthcare team established, you are going to work with them to get yourself healed. This takes some effort on your part. It also required adopting some new habits, which can be fun!

First, keep a log of the appointments you are making and the purpose of each one. I use Evernote to keep myself organized. It's just important to use something! As you progress, it may be easy to forget which doctor you'll be seeing next. If you feel that there is nothing to discuss at your appointment, cancel it.

You'll want to bring questions with you. This means that you need to be prepared for the appointments you are making. Since I use Evernote, I add to my list of questions for each doctor. I like Evernote since I have it on my phone and I always have it with me.

If your doctor uses an online system to for your medical record, great! It's an easy way to schedule appointments, get lab results and most importantly, communicate with your doctors. On a side note, I was able to use the inbox feature of the online system MyChart (the online medical system one of my doctors uses) to email to my endocrinologist and propose reducing medications based on the vitals that my naturopath had done that day. This was a great way to communicate without having to go in for an appointment!

During the appointment ask for printouts or a copy of anything the doctor documents or writes down. Even if you have access to an online system that has the information the doctor is looking at, ask for it. This will show them that you want to understand what is going on with your body and that you are serious about getting better.

Create a place where you keep all of your information from the appointments. I use both a paper folder and Evernote. I just take a picture of various documents and file them in Evernote. I also have a big folder with all of the information, so I can track the results and my progress.

It's also a good idea to bring someone with you to your appointment to be another set of ears. It takes a lot of concentration to be able to listen to all that the doctors are saying, remember the answers and ask the questions that you have. Since the appointments are usually very short and sometimes rushed, you want to make sure you are not missing any information. It helps me relax knowing that someone else is hearing what I'm hearing. In addition, you can talk over your appointment, your thoughts and feelings about it with that person who came with you.

If you are not able to bring someone with you, try voice recording the appointment. I use the voice recorder on my phone and I ask the doctor beforehand if it's ok for me to record the appointment. They are usually agreeable to this.

Part of your treatment will probably include taking medication or supplements. At first taking medication on a regular basis was a foreign concept for me. It was hard to remember what to take when. Put sticky note on your mirror and on your fridge. Keep a bottle with just a few pills that you take in your purse or your car, that way you'll always have some with you if you forget to take it.

In order to remember to take what you are prescribed, try setting an alarm in your phone to go off every day at a particular time to remind you to take them. Your phone always remembers!

As you are making these changes, be kind to yourself. Try not to expect all these changes to happen overnight. Listen to that inner voice and if you need help with that, join the community of like-minded people who can give you encouragement.

Chapter 7 – Tests to Ask For

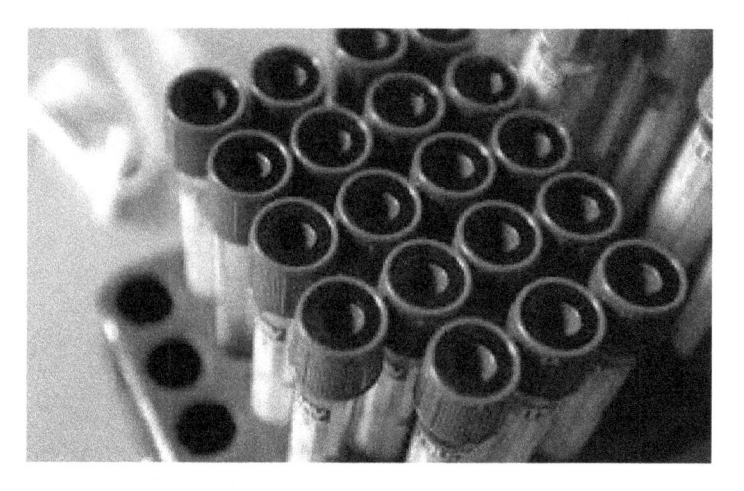

Now you're rockin' and rollin'! You've got your healthcare team, you have systems in place to remember to take your medication and supplements. Now, it's time to get some data to figure out where your body is and how to get things back into balance.

There are a number of tests that your endocrinologist and naturopath will order for you. Each has a different purpose. Remember that many of the tests your endocrinologist will have you do are to confirm the disease you have, which helps them treat you. Meanwhile, the tests your naturopath orders are to determine the status and health of your various body systems. They are trying to get you back to health.

In order to understand the blood tests, we've got to understand what the function of the thyroid is. The major thyroid hormone created by the thyroid gland is thyroxine, which is also called T4. The T4 is converted to triiodothyronine, called T3 by the removal of an iodine atom. This occurs mainly in the liver and in certain tissues where T3 acts, such as in the brain.

The amount of T4 produced by the thyroid gland is controlled by another hormone, which is made in the pituitary gland, called thyroid stimulating hormone called TSH.

The amount of TSH that the pituitary sends into the blood stream depends on the amount of T4 that the pituitary sees. If the pituitary notices very little T4, then it produces more TSH to tell the thyroid gland to produce more T4. Once the T4 in the blood stream goes above a certain level, the pituitary's production of TSH shuts off.

The thyroid and pituitary are like a heater and a thermostat. When the heater is off and it becomes cold, the thermostat reads the temperature and turns on the heater. When the heat rises to an appropriate level, the thermostat senses this and turns off the heater. Thus, the thyroid and the pituitary, like a heater and thermostat, turn on and off.

This explains why you'll get blood tests that are looking at your T3, T4 and TSH levels.

The other tests you'll experience include:

Saliva test for Adrenal Stress Index – this measures the cortisol in the body according to our natural patterns, as well as other hormones that help regulate our body. The results will provide a good indication to issues with your adrenal glands.

Food sensitivity tests - some experts believe that the inflammation in our body may contribute to the Graves' disease. The food sensitivity test determines foods that you are sensitive to, not allergic to. There are two different types of reactions: the IgE and IgG.

- In an IgE reaction, which stands for Immunoglobulin E. mediated reaction – you get exposed to a protein in a food and your immune system is triggered to mount an IgE response. The response can be either acute (immediate) or a delayed reaction. An IgE immune response causes an allergic response like rashes, swelling, wheezing and full blown anaphylaxis.

- The IgG is a different antibody mediated reaction – it measures exposure of incompletely digested food proteins that have crossed your intestinal tract and entered the blood stream. When an indigested protein enters your blood stream, the only defense that your body has at that point is to mount an immune defense.

Hair analysis – is used to evaluate the mineral content is because many people have imbalances in various minerals that are very important to thyroid health. You cut hair from small patches from your ears down on the back of your head.

This test can reveal some of the underlying causes to your Graves' like nutritional deficiencies, mineral imbalances and heavy metal and chemical toxicity.

Chapter 8 – How to Approach Your Mind

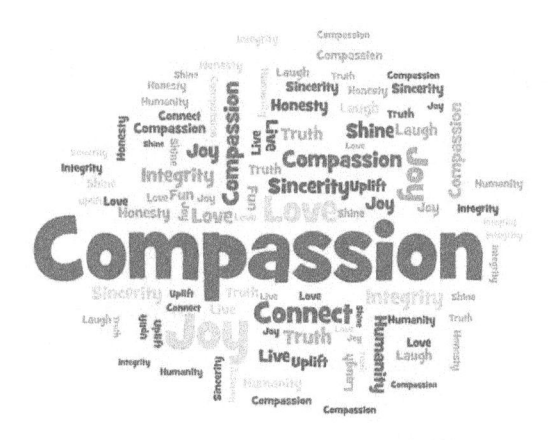

There are a few things you can do right away to start healing yourself that begin inside yourself. I want a little cartoon angel and devil sitting on my shoulders, who read my mind and tell me what to do! They would be really helpful in keeping me on track.

There is a lot of information tied to the mind-body connection. When I was following everything from the doctors perfectly and I still wasn't getting better, I felt it was time to explore other options. The literature focused on healing from the inside out beginning with the mind.

There are a lot of aspects to healing from your mind for you to explore, here are some to get you started.

Mindset

Once I complained that I had no shoes until I met a man who had no feet. That one always makes me stop and think how lucky we are. One way to understand that quote is to realize that the things that happen in your life only have the meaning that you give them. Try to see the positive side of things. Everything you experience in your life from the moment you wake up until your head hits the pillow you have a choice about the meaning you give things – choose the positive side!

Finding Fulfillment

After we make the mindset habit of realizing it's not so much the circumstances of our lives that make us happy or unhappy, but the way we see them – it's time to find fulfillment.

Fulfillment comes down to two factors:

- Love, which felt when we give happiness to others

- Compassion, which is helping others get rid of whatever is troubling them

Approaching life with love and compassion slows you down in this fast paced world. Could it be your Graves' was your body telling you to look for fulfillment?

Slow Down

Many people with Graves' just need to physically slow down. As we are trying to keep up with everything in our lives, we constantly rush and try to pack as much as possible into the day. If you have too much to do in a day, could it be that you are just not prioritizing what is important? Or do you really need to do everything? Take the time to figure out what YOU really need to do and put yourself at the top of the list!

Adopt New Beliefs

Louise Hay, author of "You Can Heal Your Life" says that thyroid function has to do with self-expression, but specifically about having my turn to express myself. The throat area is connected with our ability to speak up for ourselves and ask for what we want. You may be holding yourself back.

Here are some new beliefs that you can try to start expressing yourself.

- My body knows how to heal itself and it's doing so right now.

- I am at the center of life, and I approve of myself and all that I see.

- I move beyond old limitations and now allow myself to express freely and creatively.

With all the distractions we have in our lives today, it's hard to keep control of your mind. Now is the time to start evaluating your mind and make positive changes to heal yourself.

Chapter 9 – Healthy Habits

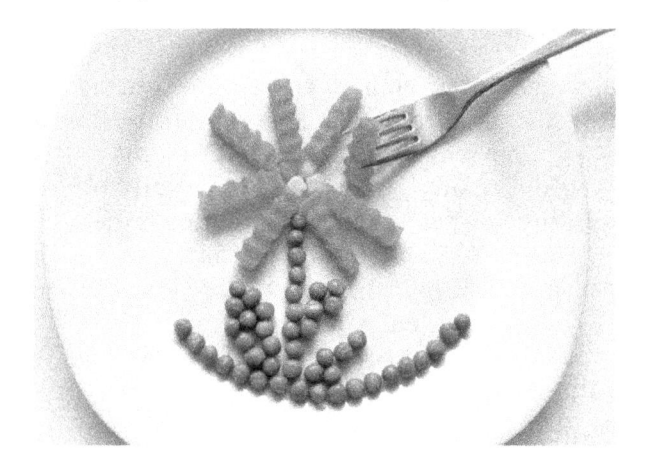

Now let's talk about your physical body and what you can do to help give your body the right canvas to heal on.

Eat right, exercise, eliminate bad stress, meditate, get enough sleep, drink plenty of water. Sounds oh-so-simple, but if we all did that we probably wouldn't be sick!

Eating Right

Graves' could be caused by an auto-immune reaction to inflammation in the body. One way to decrease the inflammation is to remove inflammatory foods from you diet. The biggest culprits are wheat, dairy, corn and soy.

I remember a friend of mine was going "gluten free", and I thought she was crazy! Gluten was a part of my breakfast, lunch, and dinner. I had no idea how I could ever do that. Fast forward a few years, and now I eat no gluten (unless I have a really weak moment!)

One approach is to remove one type of food inflammatory food completely for two weeks, then add it back into your diet and see how your body feels. You cycle through removing wheat, then dairy, then corn, then soy. For me, I've removed dairy and wheat from my diet permanently and I avoid corn and soy for the most part. I can tell if I have wheat or dairy because I get a rash on my hands.

The results from your food sensitivity tests will play a role in your diet as well. Now I eat mainly vegetables and meat. It takes a lot of planning, but is completely doable.

Stress

We are going to have stress in our lives, but it's how we deal with it that can make an impact on our immune system. Our current environment facilitates a low grade constant stress, which can wear down our bodies. Take steps to recognize the stress in your life and find ways to eliminate the constant stressors.

Exercise

Adding exercise like low to moderate cardio and strength training can be beneficial for people with Graves'. Since Graves' causes your heart to race, it's important to listen to your body. In the beginning of your healing, just focus on moving for exercise. You don't want to increase your heart rate any more than it already is.

Meditation

There are many different types of meditation that you can try. The best one for you is the one you will actually do! In the beginning, just try to sit on the floor, listen to some light music and focus on your breath for 10 minutes a day. I do this first thing in the morning and it gives me a calm clarity to carry with me the rest of the day.

Dry Brushing

Dry skin brushing can help improve the immune system by encouraging the body to release toxins on its own. You use a course brush and the bristles stimulate the blood flow and improve circulation. Try to do this once a day before you bathe.

Sleep

When I was first diagnosed with Graves' disease I was barely getting six hours of sleep a night. Now I get between 8-9 hours every night. Your body uses your sleep time to recover and prepare for the next day. Dedicating the time to sleep is important to your healing journey.

One way I've been able to implement many things in my life is to have accountability to someone else. When you tell someone else you are going to do something and you need to report back on whether you have done it or not, you are more likely to follow through and actually do what you said. This is where the Graves Recovery Camp community can help you. You post your steps and you are accountable each week to update on your progress. Just this simple step gives you the accountability to make these healthy habits a reality.

Chapter 9 – Believe You Can Heal Your Body

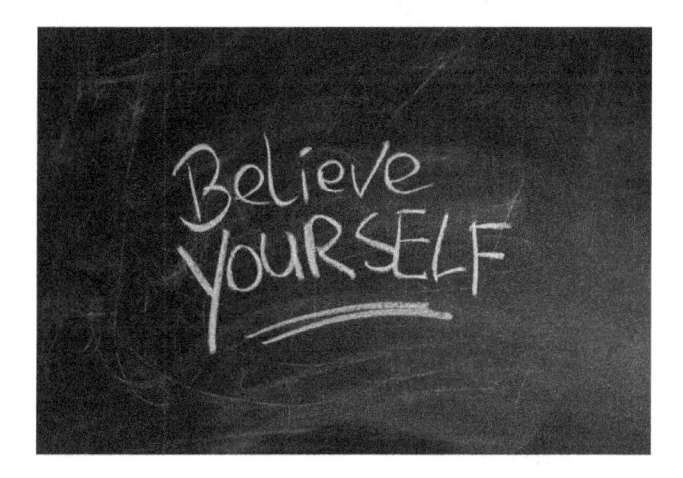

Phew!

Right now you're probably feeling a bit overwhelmed. This book is not exactly what I would consider light reading. You've just finished a full-on immersion course on Graves' disease and you should feel proud of yourself.

Being overwhelmed is actually a good thing because even though you feel like all that information is a big jumbled mess upstairs, your brain is subconsciously making connections. Right now, without you consciously doing anything. It's figuring out which treatments will be right for you. It's attracting to you the people that you need to connect with to heal. And what habits you will use to get better. All this is happening, even thought you might feel overwhelmed.

Pretty cool, right?

Your most important tools are the small habits I've given you in the book. After all this information has a chance to sink in for a day or so, go back and see how much of I you can recall. I think you'll surprise yourself!

So, what in the world should you work on first? Here's what I recommend:

1. Decide that you want to get healthy and heal your Graves' disease.

2. Create one new healthy habit a week. Don't overthink it or try to do it perfectly.

3. Write down your plan for healing. What can you start now? Go and do those things.

This book is a playbook. Don't just read it once and go on with business as usual. Keep it handy and refer to it.

Power of community

Many people who read this book need personal attention on their situation. You may need just a few simple suggestions to implement what you've just learned about.

That's what I love so much about the things you've learned in this book. They are all simple concepts that you can apply without too much effort, but the results can help you heal.

Once this books is available to millions with Graves', I know the power of community will skyrocket. The Graves' Recovery Camp community will be a movement for the healing of this disease.

Your body wants to be healthy. Try thinking of the journey of healing as a way of life to recovery. Let's tackle this together and be well!

How I can help

Living to your full POTENTIAL, by healing your Graves' Disease with natural treatment is not just a fluttering wish ANYMORE...

In case you didn't already know, that cute little butterfly gland in your neck controls a lot in your life: your health, your happiness, your energy, your relationships.

If you are picking up what I'm laying down, you're saying, "Yes, I know my thyroid needs help!" You are in the right place. Because if you've been suffering from a RUNAWAY thyroid, you'd know. You'd be dealing with a lot of these irritating issues:
- Racing heart rate
- High blood pressure

- Hair falling out
- Being mean to people you care about
- Having no patience for anyone or anything
- Feeling hot all the time
- Itching your skin raw
- Feeling tired all the time
- Having way too much energy
- Eye issues
- Bumps on your skin, especially your hands
- Brittle nails
- Losing weight
- Gaining weight
- Forgetting the simplest things
- Trying to explain the disease
- Wondering if this will turn into cancer
- Having feelings of Anxiety or Depression
- Problems sleeping

Let's get serious though

The majority of Graves' issues - being hot, skin irritations, moodiness, anxiety, weight issues stem from a less-than-healthy thyroid and, you guessed it: a thyroid that is under attack.

Think of it like this, if you tried to build two houses, one with firm cement blocks and one with styrofoam blocks, which one would be stronger?! No brainer.

In this case your thyroid is doing all it can with what it has. Most likely some foreign invader has come in through our system and taken root. The thyroid is working overtime to fight it off.

Yes. Your thyroid has gotten your attention and it's time to make some much-needed changes.

Let's build a firm foundation for our thyroid!

Because your tender butterfly gland needs some help from you.

That's why you're here.

You might be thinking, but I've tried everything, the doctors say I just need to Radiate my Thyroid. Or, I feel fine, but my blood levels are off. Or, I feel terrible and my blood levels are in-range. You don't get definitive answers, you feel like you are alone and YOU get to PAY for all of this to boot!

Trust me, I get it. I've been there.

Which is part of how I know that the solution to your thyroid problems is not removing it altogether, but it's also not throwing up your hands and saying Forget it! Even if you really want to. Frustration does that. I get it.

You might not have found the answer from your doctors, but giving up is not the answer, either. There are simple, natural ways to heal your thyroid that don't require a series of appointments, prescriptions, and expenses.

In case we haven't met yet, I'm Jen Daniele, the creator of Graves' Recovery

Camp and an advocate committed to helping people with Graves' and changing how Graves' is treated around the world.

My specialty? Guiding people to get their thyroids back to balance and their bodies back on their side. I personally know how frustrating, painful, and scary thyroid -related health issues can be. Long story short: I had Graves' disease that made me hot, extremely shaky, have a very short temper, hands shaking, hair falling out and I had legs and ankles that were raw because they itched so much. But I'm recovering, I'm healthy, and I'm here to help you feel and BE truly healthy starting from the inside out.

Because you've got so much life to live! My Graves' Recovery approach combines three areas to help you heal your Graves' #GravesRecovery4Life.

Food
What we put into our bodies are the building blocks. Nutrition impacts your thyroid. Did you know that some foods can help you heal from within? That's right. With some simple changes (and mouthwatering recipes), you can start rebuilding your body with foods that support your thyroid health goals instead of antagonizing your thyroid.

Lifestyle
Fact: no amount of food and supplements can overcome the damage that persistent stress, bad relationships, poor work environments,

negative attitudes, or lack of sleep creates. Your health depends on your habits and that goes for your thyroid health too.

Accountability
Knowing what to do and actually doing it are two different things. Getting the right healthcare team assembled, then getting the support, direction, and guidance to actually implement all the lifestyle changes - that's what you need to really make a change.

Setting the Bar
No one knew that a human could run a four minute mile until Roger Bannister ran in 1954. Now that record has been broken 18 times. Up until people knew it was possible it wasn't possible! Same thing with Graves' recovery, until people knew it was possible it wasn't possible.

There are thousands of stories of people healing their Graves' disease through lifestyle changes - that's taking care of you mind and body. Adding new ways of living to your life.

Consider the possibilities of what can happen get your food, lifestyle, and accountability right...

You become unstoppable, able to live to your best...

You start living to your potential - tackling your dreams head on with confidence and excitement, no more putting it off or waiting until you're rid of Graves'.

You have relationships with people the way you want to - close and intimate with some - warm and loving with others - all the connections are adding to your life!

You get back to having ENERGY — no more exhaustion for no reason, tiredness, slothiness, or being so tired that you can't sleep.

You are able to exercise without worry of getting your heart rate up too high, and live in your body in very active ways!

You get to the weight you want without having to battle to either keep the weight on or off.

What's more?

Your potential is limitless...

You're ready to be healthy. You're ready for more. You're ready to have the life you really want.

You're ready to become UNSTOPPABLE. And you're about to, because you're finally READY to make this commitment to YOU.

Introducing Graves' Recovery Camp
The program, community, and support

you need to get your thyroid in check and become the unstoppable person you were meant to be.

Join Now

In a nutshell, I created Graves' Recovery Camp as a way to help more people like YOU get the direction, guidance and support they really need, AND at a price they could afford. The people wanted each other. Look, it's one thing to be told what you "should" do, but it's another to have friends who GET what you are going through and hold you accountable to making the changes you really want to make.

Enter: The Campers

These people are your people, your buddies, your cheerleaders. I've learned through my experience that doing this alone is hard and grueling. You make more progress, endure longer and have people to celebrate with when you are surrounded by a tribe like-minded people, going through the same journey as you. People who truly understand the struggle and get what you're going through.

These people know the pain of being tired all the time, their hair falling out, feeling hot, being depressed and anxious at the same time. Yes, this happens to LOTS of people. One in 200 people have Graves'. And they are waiting for you inside Graves' Recovery Camp.

WHAT IS Graves' Recovery Camp REALLY?

Graves' Recovery Camp is a membership community that provides its members with the Graves' Recovery Camp Blueprint, discussion forums, member calls, community, and ongoing group support.

But Graves' Recovery Camp is more than a program, it's a movement. Where people take charge of their thyroid health, and lives, together.

What You'll Get When You Become a Camper:

- Graves' Recovery Camp Blueprint - A collection of video courses with handouts that leads you step by step through the path to recovery and help you adopt the new habits.
- Twice-A-Month Member Calls - Imagine being able to get all of your thyroid questions answered AND hear from others LIVE on the phone. You'll get to do that twice a month as a Camper.
- Steps to Find Your Healthcare Team - Defining who you need on your team, exploring the the process of selecting and interviewing the professionals to make sure they are a fit for you. Questionnaires to ask them to make sure you have the right people.
- Motivational Challenges - Ranging from sleep to meditation challenges, these challenges are led by yours truly

with additional livestreams and these have been designed to keep you on point with your protocol.
- Thyroid Affirmations - Directing your subconscious through specific affirmations targeting your health and thyroid health.
- Meditations - Focused on finding the peace and calm to heal your thyroid from within.
- The Campers - Your Community of Supportive People – your cheerleaders, your people, and friends. You don't know them yet, but soon you'll ask yourself how you EVER tried to do any of this without them. Trust me.
- Cooking Tutorials - You'll get step-by-step instruction on how to tackle this meal plan head on. Learn even how to adjust the recipes to your taste or to accommodate them based on any food sensitivities you may have.

Join Now
It's less than a gym membership, less than your daily Caffeine habit (right?!), less than a mani/pedi, and about a million TIMES the value of your lifelong health, IF you can even put a price on your health. Can you put a price on all you're going through? I didn't think so.

THIS IS YOUR HEALTH WE'RE TALKING ABOUT!

How to Become a Camper...
Just go to www.gravesrecoverycamp.com to join.

You can use any major credit card to complete your purchase.

Once you submit payment, you'll get an immediate WELCOME email with all of your log-in details to access your content and join the Campers online!
You'll also get a welcome video to help you get started in the Community. Whoo hoo! You'll start healing that butterfly gland, getting the support you need and you'll get your life back! Join Now.

You might be saying to yourself... "but I've already tried so many things. How do I know THIS will work?"
First, let me say: "I get it. I've been there"
Most of the people who start this program are in the exact same place as you right now.

They've been to tons of doctors, they've been put on an antithyroid medication and a beta blockers. They feel alone because they don't have anyone to really talk to about it. Doctors spend such little time with them. And,
They've been told that removing their thyroid through radio-active iodine is the only way to get better. But, that gives them an 80% chance of going Hypothyroid.

Here is how Graves' Recovery Camp is different...

You'll get more access and more personalized attention.

Since this is the first time Graves' Recovery Camp is being offered, you'll be getting special one-on-one attention that is available before there are 100's in the Community. It's the best time to get help and support.

Graves' Recovery Camp is NOT a one-size-fits-all program.

It's customized to YOU. When you join, you'll get to explore the lessons in the Graves' Recovery Camp Blueprint. You'll ask your questions. You'll be putting in your accountability, what you are actually going to do. And I will follow up with you to make sure you are taking those steps. It's amazing the action we will take when we know we have to report back to someone cares about what we are doing. This program is here to help you.

You'll only get out of it what you put into it. Graves' Recovery Camp is not about FAST results, it's about revamping your health. It's a natural approach based on a holistic approach to the human body. All that said, you have to commit to the program and do the work in order to heal.

Any other Questions?
How do I pay for the program and what happens after I sign up?
Awesome! By signing up, you'll be registering

yourself as an official "Camper". You will be billed each month on the same day each month. Because it takes time and consistency to see improvements in your health, I recommend that you commit yourself to the program for at least three months. Although, once you're in the community, I don't think you'll ever wanna leave! All that said, you're free to cancel at any time.

Will I receive anything via mail?
NOPE. This is a fully online program – accessible worldwide! From your phone, laptop, tablet, or desktop computer! After you purchase you'll get an email giving you immediate access to your membership site with your user name and password. You can hop into the forums and start asking questions!

How long do I have to stay in Graves' Recovery Camp to see results?
This varies from person to person. It depends on your case and your commitment. I've seen people get better in one month, and others, like me, it's taken years. Best thing to do is start doing all you can to give your body the clean slate to heal.

What is your cancellation policy?
Boy, oh boy! We haven't even started yet! ;) JK (as my kids say). It's easy to cancel anytime. You can do so through the account settings within the Membership area. Because I want you to give this program your ALL, I ask that you commit yourself for three months

minimum.

How about refunds?
This program is billed monthly so you can come and go as it suits you and your finances. However, we do not provide refunds. As long as you cancel your membership, you will not be billed for any future months.

What if I am too old? Too young? Is this program for ME?
YES. This program is for you. Graves' is just the way your body is yelling to you, "Please take care of me!" Whether you're in your 20s or 60s, or have Graves' or have it at bay. Graves' Recovery Camp was designed for ALL people with Graves' – we have Campers of all shapes, sizes, ages, and lifestyles and it's working for them. So, let's get started on your healing!

I'm so tired of trying to heal my Graves' disease. What if this is just "too hard"?
I hear you. There are days I have too where I want to say, Forget It! I'm just going to give up! But then, I come to my senses and realize, this is the ONLY Alternative. I don't want to continue on a downward spiral with my health. I can't sugar coat this - #nosugar. Committing to Graves' Recovery Camp will not be easy. YOU have to do the work and commit to the program in order to see the results. Ask yourself, are you worth it? Is your life worth it? I know the answer is a resounding - YES.

The truth is that only YOU know what your health, life, and well-being is worth to you. I'm simply here to help you get there, and this is your official invitation to take a step in the right direction.

What if I have more questions? Can I get access to you?
Definitely! Our twice a month Member calls are designed just for that – so you can get all of your questions answered right away! In addition, I'm very active in our online community.

One last thing...
   Look, I've been in the "Valleys" of life too. I thought I was losing my mind when Graves' was in full force for me. I was irritable, extremely uncomfortable in my own skin. I had to take care of my family, work full time, add all kinds of new practices to my life, and develop a new business at all hours in order to make it work. I built this because I was sick of seeing how quickly people have their thyroids taken out, it's an irreversible situation that can leave you with lifelong issues. I know I could have used the support and direction to make my path a lot easier. Remember that sometimes, no matter how hard it is, change is necessary.
   Your potential is limitless. You CAN heal your body, you CAN love your life, you CAN feel like you can live to YOUR potential. What I know from my own story is this: your body is telling you to shape up. It's your wake up call. It will only let you

continue to work against it, for so long. Then it will start telling you LOUDER that what you are doing is NOT good for it – and even though it's Graves' right now, it could be other chronic issues in the future. I'm not trying to scare you, I just want you to wake up and shape up.

What I MOST want is for you is to take action NOW, before anything more happens.

You owe it to yourself to do something now.

YOU'VE GOT THIS.

Thank you so much!

I hope you've enjoyed this book as much as I loved writing it for you. I can't thank you enough for your continued support of The Graves Recovery Camp blog and everything I do. I appreciate each and every one of you for taking your time to read this, and if you have an extra second, I would love to hear what you think about it. Please visit: http://www.gravesrecoverycamp.com/

Or if you'd rather say hello on Twitter, I'm @jendaniele. Join in on the conversations going on right now on my Facebook page too!

Thank you so much for reading and I wish for you a healthy life!

Jen Daniele

References

Bankova, Svetla. www.gravesdiseasecure.com, 2016

Blum, Susan. The Immune System Recovery Plan, New York: Scribner 2013

Flanigan, Jessica. The Loving Diet, New York: Post Hill Press, 2015

Hay, Louise. You Can Heal Your Life, California: H Life Styles, 1999

Moore, Elaine. www.Elaine-moore.com, 2015

Moore, Elaine. Graves' Disease, A Practical Guide, North Carolina: McFarland & Company, 2001

Osansky, Eric. www.naturalendocrinesolutions.com, 2016

Thyroid Disease Manager, www.thyroidmanager.org, 2016

www.ingramcontent.com/pod-product-compliance
Lightning Source LLC
LaVergne TN
LVHW041244230325
806616LV00039B/1267